Time to Live, Time to Die

D0898969

Time to Live, Time to Die

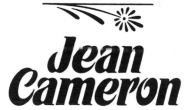

Jean Cameron

**Forewords by
Elisabeth Kübler-Ross
and Balfour Mount**

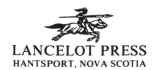

LANCELOT PRESS
HANTSPORT, NOVA SCOTIA

TIME TO LIVE AND TIME TO DIE

Published under title *For All That Has Been* by
Macmillan Publishing Co., Inc., New York, 1982
Published by Lancelot Press Limited, 1987
by arrangement with author and original publisher.

Second printing July 1988
Third printing March 1990
Fourth printing June 1991
ISBN 0-88999-333-5
Designed by Robert Pope

All rights reserved. No part of this book may be reproduced in any form without written permission of the publishers except brief quotations embodied in critical articles or reviews.

LANCELOT PRESS LIMITED, Hantsport, Nova Scotia
Office and production facilities situated on Hwy. No. 1,
1/2 mile east of Hantsport, N.S.

*To Louise — the constant friend,
without whom none of this would have been possible*

—Night is drawing nigh—
For all that has been — Thanks!
To all that shall be — Yes!
DAG HAMMARSKJÖLD

Contents

Foreword

I HAVE BEEN waiting for this book for several years. Not that there are not many books on the market that describe personal suffering, the facing and struggle of a terminal illness, the growth that can come out of it — but this is a different story and one that must be shared.

I met Jean many years ago in Montreal, in the context of my own work with death and dying, my worldwide lectures on the topic, and, last but not least, the opening of my favorite palliative care unit at Royal Victoria Hospital in Montreal. I meet up to 15,000 people a week and see so many health professionals and patients that I rarely remember a name. But I always remember faces and one or two special people in each crowd. Jean was one of them, a sensitive, almost delicate lady with a heart of gold and an intuitive understanding of human beings. I think, looking back over the years, she always represented a model of faith, trust, and love all encompassed in one human being who has gone through the tumbler of life and emerged polished like a diamond.

Jean's story is a part of her life, the part that brought her to the bedside of those faced with a terminal illness and her role in helping them to live to the best of their potential. It shares with us the awareness of her own illness, the changing role from help-giver to help-receiver, and through it all, it shows that someone who has this faith and inner strength can teach and share and help to the end.

When she says, "When a person looks at you and loves, you are no longer ugly and unclean with disease, and each day seems a precious gift to be cherished and savored to the full," Jean is the one who has faced so many needy and desperate patients with that loving look, and she now harvests, in a small way, the love she has given and continues to give.

It was her pride to accept the responsibility of her own reaction to the illness, the treatment, pain, little deaths, and many losses until this last control was also threatened when brain metastasis was verified. She faced this ultimate challenge with the same determination and courage and emerged free of fear and guilt, remembering the lives she touched and the lives that touched hers — a constant giving and receiving of unconditional love without claims and expectations. When her bells ring, she will know that she has been a gift to this world and that this world is a better place because she has lived.

This book should be read by many health care givers and those who face a terminal illness. It will give them strength, courage, and faith that even the seemingly unfair and dreadful windstorms of life ultimately are responsible for beauty and wisdom. Jean and her book are full of both.

ELISABETH KÜBLER-ROSS

Foreword

FROM OUR earliest association, in 1974, Jean Cameron has stood out as someone special. Ernest Hemingway would have said that Jean has "guts," for she has indeed exhibited "grace under pressure." Prevented by ill health from working full time in her professional capacity as a social worker, Jean turned her attention to clinical research. She joined the fledgling Royal Victoria Hospital Palliative Care Service in its days of infancy and quickly earned a reputation as a capable, sensitive, and perceptive consultant. Her efforts on behalf of bereaved family members were tireless. A full 123 pages of the original Palliative Care Service Pilot Project Report were written by Jean, documenting the results of her studies. Her thoughtful intervention and analysis of bereavement problems have been cited by Dr. Colin Murray Parkes of the London Hospital as a significant contribution to the field of bereavement research.

In May 1975, only five months after commencement of the PCS, Jean learned that she had cancer. Her response was characterized by a resilience born out of her prolonged experience with suffering. For years Jean had appreciated the writings of Viktor Frankl. His observation that the last of human freedoms is our ability to choose our response whatever the circumstance, struck a chord in her. Facing progressive disease herself, she became preoccupied by the needs of others. Months passed into years, and as the ravages of tumour advancement took their toll, Jean simply seemed to grow in stature. Her own suffering gave her a special place in the hearts of the patients and families she cared for.

In the pages of this book the reader has the unusual opportunity of experiencing with Jean the trials and tribulations of advancing malignant disease. Many of the problems she faced are common among cancer patients. For Jean, however, there was an extra dimension of complexity because of her status as a health care professional. She was friend as well as patient, care giver as well as recipient of care. Tensions rose in spite of the best efforts of all concerned. Those involved found themselves facing the same dilemmas, the same strained relationships that confront our patients and their families on a daily basis. Throughout these difficult months Jean continued to grow in understanding, patience, and grace. For her it has been a process of opening to others, to herself, and to her God. Jean Vanier once described prayer as "the opening of the cup of our being." Jean's life has become a prayer.

In *Time to Live, Time to Die* we encounter a refreshing unevenness in style that reflects the intensity with which these pages were written. We pass from the tightly written, superbly descriptive prose describing her encounters with those in need of help, to the almost painfully detailed analytical recounting of her own bruised feelings and anger as she experiences the stresses and frustrations of inadequate care. Jean's honesty and sensitivity to others cannot but touch us and remind us that in spite of recent improvements in terminal care there are indeed "miles to go before we sleep."

In recent years Jean has felt increasingly able to share her experiences and insights with others. She has participated in television programs for Canadian, American, British, and Italian networks, held countless interviews, and lectured to thousands. Now she gives us this book. Her impact on all of us was summed up for me in the face of a first year McGill medical student who stopped me in a hospital corridor five months after hearing Jean speak about suffering and bereavement. Her perspective, she said with great feeling, has been permanently altered! These pages are a rare and personal look at a remarkable woman. It is my privilege to claim Jean Cameron as my colleague, teacher, and friend.

BALFOUR M. MOUNT, M.D., FRCS. (C)
Director Palliative Care Service,
Professor of Surgery, McGill University

Acknowledgments

I SHOULD LIKE to thank all those whose love and support made it possible for me to write this little book. Many people helped in all kinds of ways. I hope they will understand and realize my gratitude although I cannot mention all their names.

I am especially grateful to Dr. Colin Murray Parkes for his encouragement and help through all the ups and downs of the past few years; to Dr. Ina Ajemian, Dr. Balfour Mount, and the staff of the Palliative Care Service for their continuing friendship and care; and to Dr. Peter Hacker for his unfailing love and support.

I owe a special debt to the great teachers — Dr. Elisabeth Kübler-Ross, Dame Cicely Saunders, and Father Benedict Vanier — whom I have been privileged to know.

I also want to say a special thank you to Ramona Ibbotson for the hours of typing and other help so kindly given.

But perhaps most of all I am grateful to all those people who opened their hearts and shared their times of sorrow, pain, and joy, reflected in these pages with my own.

1
The Last Night

The storm of the last night
Has crowned this morning
With golden peace.[1]

ONE GROWS accustomed to the spread of cancer. New symptoms appear, and when they persist or increase one mentions them, tests are made, and results confirm suspicions. The disease seems to travel on relentlessly in my body — breasts, neck, shoulder, spine, hip, lung. One day it must surely overcome some vital organ. Meantime, the preoccupation has been with learning to cope and to continue to function as each new restriction and limitation is added.

I used to say, "I cannot alter the course of this disease and I cannot understand it or the reason I have it. It is beyond my control." Just occasionally, I understand how I should use some of the experience, perhaps to help another. But the reason the disease is present has never seemed all that important. It is beyond my comprehension and I do not expect to understand it. The important thing it to accept. What I felt I could control was my own reaction to it: how I cope, how I live with it, and perhaps how I die with it. This I felt was my task.

Viktor Frankl expressed this clearly when he wrote, "Everything can be taken from man but one thing, the last of the human freedoms — to choose one's attitude in any given set of circumstances, to choose one's own way."[2] This is what I had hoped to be able to do until the end of my life. This would be my task and my "freedom."

A few weeks ago, however, new symptoms could no longer be denied (headaches, nausea, a feeling of pressure as if my head might burst, vision blurred and clouded over). All told me that something was happening, and I didn't want to admit to any of it. The fear of brain involvement has always been present but firmly pushed aside as too painful to contemplate. I could talk easily about death and even my fears of choking or of intolerable pain or all the other fears, but never this, the greatest fear of all. The development of brain metastases was something too awful to face.

The possibility of changes in psychological functioning had always seemed to me much more threatening than any of the physical changes that disease has brought. To know how I am acting or reacting and to be able to control this seemed extremely important.

Brain metastases have been confirmed and may take away this one crucial part of myself that is left. Until now, I have known if I was causing too much stress, worry, or exhaustion to those who care for me, and I could alter arrangements and ease the burdens. But psychological impairment could alter all this and I might not understand or even realize the changes. I might become irritable, complaining, unreasonable, demanding, or might unwittingly hurt the very people I love the most. Ability to recognize the true situation is no longer a certainty. But the love is even stronger and with it the desire not to cause pain.

Two weeks ago I could not have written this chapter. My peace was shaken. My immediate reaction to the diagnosis was that I would tell no one. A kind of panic swept over me. It seemed to me that if people had been able to attribute what had seemed normal reactions of justifiable anger at certain situations to the effects of the disease before, how much more likely would they be able to attribute everything with which they disagreed to an improperly functioning brain. How easy it would be.

I felt an almost paranoid reaction — everyone would be watching and looking for signs of the deteriorating mind. Gone would be my hopes of functioning or of being treated as normal. I would avoid telling anyone except those few people who are very close to me and whom I could trust above all

20

others. Subsequently, I realized the obligation to explain the situation to those people for whom I still do a little work, to give them freedom for the painful task of telling me if I can no longer function adequately or become incapable of useful contribution to the task.

Slowly and gradually, then, came the realization that nothing is really as terrible as the fear of it. I know now that it is possible to accept and somehow to cope even with this. I believe that the people who love me will have the strength and courage to arrange for placement if I should become too much of a burden. I know that they will not let me or themselves down by failing in the difficult final task if it should become necessary.

Of course, none of this may ever come to pass. The experts say that the effects of the brain metastases may be insignificant and that it is likely that some other vital organ will succumb to the disease and bring about the final collapse. Certainly for the present the physical symptoms have been relieved by medication. But no one can be sure.

Painfully and slowly I have been allowed to climb over this last hurdle, the greatest fear of all, and it is gone. The essential trust and faith remain; I know now how strong they are and whence they come. I am even more conscious of the importance of the love and support of those who really care and understand.

I am at peace and each day seems even more precious. I work a little harder, wanting to share and proclaim the truth as I see it and wanting to leave behind a simple testimony to the people who are special in my life.

I lie here looking out of my window. The sun shines and the squirrels and birds are squabbling and chattering as they scramble for nuts on my windowsill, knocking over the plant pots in their enthusiasm.

Slowly I am learning to accept the humility of doing and giving less and less, and receiving more. Physical strength diminishes but a special kind of joy and peace comes to fill the void.

I listen to music on my precious tapes. It raises my spirits far above the pain and suffering, and sometimes, very rarely, it releases a flood of helpless weeping until I am empty, restored again by its beauty and tranquility to the calm and peace of its healing. Life is good: the happiness is real. I give thanks "for all that has been" and now I *can* say "Yes" to whatever lies ahead. I lie here waiting, but for what? Dare I say hoping? (My trusty English dictionary never defines that word as denial.)

At any moment the telephone may ring with a call from someone who needs to talk, to share a time of pain or sorrow. I am ready to use whatever strength remains if it is asked. And if there is to be no more and my task is done, my bag is packed. I do not fear this journey.

A short time ago an eminent psychiatrist, whom I am privileged to know as a friend, spent some hours with me. After he left he climbed to the top of a nearby mountain, and, as he stood looking down from the summit, he shared his thoughts in a few lines on a postcard that he mailed to me the next day. He wrote of the essential oneness of all creation, saying, "You and I and the rivers and the earth are, perhaps, only separated by an illusion of aloneness. Only the trivial is transient." I think I understand now what he meant.

2
The Call

The door is open: oceans and hills all point to the road.
The night near your head will stand silent
For death is a call to the wayfarer.[3]

IT WAS very quiet in the little room, the silence broken only by the sounds of quick, shallow breathing. Sitting beside her husband's bed, Mrs. Grey watched and waited as his life slowly ebbed.

When she turned, the tears welling in her eyes, I remembered the words she had spoken just a few days before. "You know, the real sadness of dying comes just before the end. You can go so far with people you love. You can share and live with them through all that happens for a long time and even during the last illness. But then you gradually find that you are being left behind. You realize that they are going away on their own somewhere. You can't go with them. You are losing them. They are dying and you are being left alone."

Looking back, remembering, it seems a short time ago that I first walked down the corridor and into the hospital ward for dying cancer patients, hoping to understand, eager to help. A kaleidoscope of people and faces comes to mind. They take shape, some old like Mr. Grey, some young like Philip, but all of them dying, preparing for that last journey.

I remember the day when Mr. Grey was brought into the ward, his face ashen with pain and fatigue. He seemed not to understand where he was going or what was happening. He really didn't care anymore.

Mrs. Grey, hurrying along beside the stretcher, looked tired, strained, and anxious. She was exhausted by the months of trying to care for her husband at home. Later, she would describe her feelings on that day.

They had fought this sickness for so long together. Was she really now giving up the fight? He had begged to be allowed to stay at home. He hated the hospital. But the pain was terrible and they were both exhausted. Had she really let him down by bringing him to this place? Here everybody dies. What dread lay in those words. She knew now that by coming here she was finally admitting that he too would die.

She watched as gentle hands helped him into a warmed bed and then she looked around, guardedly, cautiously. The faces seemed friendly and relaxed. Patients seemed alert, even happy. They chatted. Some were plainly busy. She heard laughter down the hall. Could it be that all of them were really dying?

A few days later, Mr. Grey was lying awake in his bed. His pain had been relieved. Refreshed by a long sleep, he was alert and comfortable once more. On the shelf beside him was a vase of freshly picked garden flowers.

I looked at the wizened face, at the hollow eyes, penetratingly blue. A flicker of a smile appeared as I sat down beside him. He whispered, "I know I'm not going to get better." No words were needed. I touched his hand and we were quiet. A tear rolled down a furrowed cheek. In a stronger, pleading voice he said, "But don't you see, I only just retired — worked all those extra years to provide us with more comfort and security. I fixed up the house, tiled the kitchen myself, paid off the mortgage. I have this garden. You see those flowers on the window sill? My wife brought them in. I grew them. I know she tries to keep them weeded for me now but it is hard for her, and she comes here each day to be with me.

"I know I'm old now and people think it's not so bad for me to die. But you see, there are still those hopes and dreams that I have, simple things of life that belong to retirement. Now there is time to sit in the yard with my wife, to smoke my pipe, to watch my garden grow. Smell those pinks there. Nice, aren't they? It's almost time to set out the nicotina — lovely sweet smell in the summer evenings.

"Do you understand? I still want to get better and live. It could all be so good now. And I have all those memories to think about, my wife and I, if only we could have a little more time together."

But time was running out for Mr. Grey just as it did for every patient on that ward. Some were ready and some were not.

Across the hall from Mr. Grey, a tiny, frail form lies propped on the pillows. The eyes flutter open. "How is it today?" But you already know, sensing the quiet peace. She whispers, "There's no pain — just very tired." The eyes close.

Softly and swiftly a young woman with anxious eyes comes in, and two small children clamber up to kiss the face that's wreathed in smiles and new-found strength. There is eager chatter about new-born kittens and things the children have seen and done. She listens happily, but soon fatigue becomes exhaustion. "Grannie is very tired now." The pair are led away to draw pictures in the lounge. The daughter sits quietly holding her mother's hand as she lies with closed eyes and shallow breath.

Some time later the children tiptoe back with the pictures they have made for Gran of the house where they live, the cows in the neighbour's field. They watch quietly as the bright scenes are carefully taped to the wall in front of Gran's bed where she will see them and be reminded of the visit when she wakes up.

The quiet returns, and then softly, as if to herself, she whispers, "They've all been so good to me. They took me to live with them and tried to make me feel it was my home too. But it's not the same. It will never be the same without my Jack. But I'll soon be with him now. Oh, yes, it's been a good life. I've no regrets — just tired, so very tired."

Palliative care — so many people, so many different kinds of pain cry out for relief. There are those who have caring families, and those who have no families, and those whose families don't seem to care at all.

A young woman wrote:

Do not come
  Rushing to my grave
    Crying your heart out
      When I die
Your tears will be a lie

Only the grass will grow
  Tall and strong
    As they water it
For me they will have no merit

You should have cared
  For me a bit
    While I was around
      To be touched
You could have done so much
For me — with so little —
    Now . . . let the grass wither.[4]

An old man was brought into the men's ward who lay in silent resignation. One day he said, "They do what they want with me now. I have no say. There is nothing left. I'm just a useless burden. Family you say? Yes, they are here now. They've come, just for a little while, waiting for me to die. They are all young and strong and they're impatient to be rid of me. Then they'll be able to hurry off again on their separate ways. They think I don't know. But I see it there, written in their faces. Eyes that will not meet mine. Impatient gestures that say 'Hurry up and get it over with.' I never thought that it would come to this. Well, it won't be long now. I'm not hungry any more. It's better not to eat. Pain? My pain is loneliness. But it's all finished now. I'm through with living. No one really cares. Perhaps I can just sleep now in this place. That will be a good way to go." He turned his face to the wall.

But in that place, he, like the simple little man down the hall who had nowhere to go and who stayed so long, found that people cared about him after all.

There was a little man who was small of stature but big of heart. He had no home. No one wanted him. He was slow to understand: some called him simple. He wanted desperately to be needed. He loved to help on the ward. With careful pride in each humble task he helped staff and patients alike whenever he could. He was an outcast, yet he still loved his fellow human beings. Above all he loved his God.

One day his friend and roommate died. It was a peaceful death and Paul was there at the end, mutely watching from the corner of the room with tear-filled eyes. When it was over he stood by his friend's bed in respectful silence. Then he turned to the weeping widow and asked if he might say a prayer. He stood there quietly and reverently, then bowed his head and said his simple prayer — in French.

Long afterward the lady was heard to say, "That little man — I didn't understand a single word of what he was saying. But it was the most beautiful and heart-warming moment when he said that prayer. I was more touched by that and more grateful than for anything else that happened."

A few days later this lady came back to visit Paul, even though it was hard for her, especially so because someone else was in her husband's bed.

Paul was with us for a long time before he died. These lines came to mind as a simple epitaph:

Beneath this tree
The shadow of a shade
A little humble smiling man is laid.
He loved his life
Of death was not afraid
And loved his maker
'Though so strangely made.

3
Last Salutations

My last salutations are to them
Who knew me imperfect and loved me.[5]

A SPECIAL FEELING creeps into the ward at the end of the day, a kind of warmth and peace in the quiet of evening. The bustle of the day's activities is over. Many of the staff have gone home. There's little now to distract the mind. Patients settle down together, relaxed, waiting for the long night.

This is a time of quiet intimacy: time to reflect, time to think of the past and what has been, time to think of what's to come. Families have left. There is no need now to pretend or try to reassure. Some share the thoughts; some share the silence. Drawn together from so many different backgrounds and life styles, in this place they are one. Together they face the simple, universal, inescapable confrontation with death. Distressing symptoms have been relieved. Each person is cared for with warmth and understanding. They will live each day until they die, but they do not forget that they are dying.

And then, for a time, the spell is broken. Along the hall the door swings open and hurrying into the ward come the first anxious figures of those who have been at work all day. Reassured by the sight of the familiar faces they settle down to chat, sharing the news of the day's events.

But some patients, already embarked on their journey, only look back through mists. They do not ask and may not speak. They lie quietly content, sensing that the loved ones are near. There are those among the visitors who will not go home tonight.

The door swings open again and the last of the workers arrives. With a quick word of greeting to the nurses at the station, she goes straight to the room where her husband is waiting. With a sad smile she embraces him and settles quietly at his side. He is a man of few words, and they sit together now as they have for so many years at home, silent, content just to be together.

For a while before he came here the pain had been bad. Now it was eased. But every day he grew weaker. For two and a half years they had fought the cancer together and even a short time ago they had still bluffed and pretended to each other that they had hopes each knew to be unreal.

But Mrs. Macdonald had always known and said that honesty and truthfulness to themselves and to each other had been one of the deepest commitments and greatest strengths of their marriage. The evening came when she finally managed to blurt out that she knew he couldn't get better. Mr. Macdonald just took her hand and held her close. A great burden had been lifted from him. There was no need to try and pretend anymore. But when, a few days later, he tried to talk about her future plans it was just too much, too soon. With tears streaming down her cheeks she ran from the room. He understood her pain and asked no more. Now each day's hopes are for the quiet evening together. She sits there beside him silently knitting.

In the next room a young man sits talking to his mother. On the table beside him all kinds of delicacies are laid out. The mother picks up each dish in turn. She coaxes, pleads with him, begs him to try and eat. He murmurs that the sight of food sickens him. She does not listen. Desperately, anxiously, she persists, trying to sustain life by the one means she knows. This is her son. He must, he will, eat to live. "Of course you can if you really try. This is all your favourite food. You must keep up your strength. You *can* get well. You can't give up. Come now, only try!" From all the pent-up emotion — the broken engagement, the fears and the pain — anger and frustration spill out, channelled into fury against his piteous mother. "For God's sake don't you realize it's no use now? It's all too late." She does not hear.

Across the hall in the women's ward a simple working woman, now frail and weak, feebly lifts her hand in welcome to her handsome grandson. But then she cries out in despair, "Why does God keep me alive? I am useless. Don't look at me; I cannot even comb my hair now." The tall young man looks down at her with a tender smile. "Well now, I guess you just have to wait your turn until God is ready. Useless? Do you forget all those years when you worked so hard and scrimped and saved for the family? You did so many things for all of us. Do you think we don't remember? Surely you have earned a little rest now. And you know, you did one thing in your life that no one else ever could." "What, what was that?" "Why, no one else was ever able to be my grandmother. And you, you are such a special grandmother." Eyes light up. Proud eyes gaze at this wonderful person, her grandson. His few simple words have given her a reason for her life and a reason to be able to let go.

Peals of laughter echo down the corridor. Mr. O'Malley has dulled all his pain with a bottle of brandy and now he sits with his friends at the card table, the bottle placed beside him, ready to be shared with any willing passerby. A short time ago his wife came in. "Where's Buster?" he asked, and the little mongrel dog leaped onto his bed, an ecstatic, wriggling bundle.

The poker game goes on with frequent interruptions. Later, when he's had a few too many, Mr. O'Malley starts dancing up and down the hall singing about an Irish colleen. His merriment is infectious and others join in, the pain forgotten. Even the rather staid and proper lady visiting next door succumbs to his charm and joins in a lively dance. Some weeks afterward, now widowed, alone in her room she remembers and smiles. "I couldn't help laughing. Although they were all so sick they could still have such fun."

Ten o'clock now and some have already drifted off to sleep. Families begin to slip away. Mrs. Macdonald packs up her knitting and prepares to leave. Mrs. O'Malley calls to Buster, "Time to go." The women meet in the hall and walk along together. They pause at a doorway and call goodnight to Mrs. Smith. She is going to stay tonight. As they start to go each wonders how long it will be before her own turn comes to stay.

Quietly they walk along the hall together, past yet another door. Alone in her room, Mrs. Brown is carefully making lists. She will stock the freezer with her husband's favourite steaks, lay in supplies of the sheets that are on sale, order some more of his shirts, leave enough of everything to tide him over those first difficult months. She will leave her house in order. Mrs. Macdonald and Mrs. O'Malley stop to bid her goodnight.

At the end of the hall, with solemn bow, Paul stands proudly holding open the door to let the ladies pass. After a special word to Paul, as they leave Mrs. O'Malley is saying, "It's like part of your own family in there, all in it together, all helping each other. You know, it seems such a safe place somehow."

That is the remarkable thing about that ward. All those dying people do feel, strangely, "safe."

4
Fear

Your shadow at morning striding behind you
Or your shadow at evening rising to meet you;
I will show you fear in a handful of dust.

T.S. ELIOT[6]

I HAD SPENT some months helping in the ward for dying patients, sitting with and listening and talking to people who were in the last stages of their illness. They talked about their experiences, the cancer, their fears, their lives, the people they loved and would leave behind, the hopes that remained, and, sometimes, how it felt to die.

And then — I remember the day very clearly — I discovered a small lump in a breast. It did not seem very significant or alarming at the time; I had had this kind of thing before. But since I happened to have a doctor's appointment that afternoon I decided to mention it, just in case. The doctor's examination revealed ominous signs, and arrangements were made immediately for consultation with a surgeon the next morning.

I went back to the hospital ward that evening after the visit to the doctor and spent some hours with the patients and their families. I remember sitting quietly at a bedside, while in the back of my mind a voice seemed to keep saying, "This can't be true — not me — not now, just when I am so involved in this work. I'm needed here." Suddenly the thought came into my mind for the first time: could I be going to end up in one of these beds?

This was the beginning of my cancer. After surgery and during chemotherapy I asked if there was some way in which I could continue to help in the work of the hospital ward. As a result, my bereavement work by telephone began. Later, feeling that useful and helpful information was emerging from the conversations, I began to write about it.

Because I was thinking a lot about those people and trying to help them, I realized how much I was really helping myself. I was often able to forget my nausea and discomfort. The work was totally absorbing. At this time I looked forward to recovery and hoped and planned to return to a more active role in the hospital as soon as I had regained strength.

I began to learn and understand many things more clearly. The theories and words heard and read became realities that I could feel; no longer was I trying to share the trials of cancer from a healthy distance.

One of the first realizations was the implication of this disease. Having had several life-threatening cardiovascular crises prior to the cancer, I noticed an interesting difference in my own reaction to this new disease. Whereas I had never hesitated to say that I had had rheumatic fever, endocarditis, a myocardial infarction, or whatever it was when asked, for some reason I was hesitating to say, "I have cancer."

Deep down I realized the stigma that is attached to this disease. When people ask about your illness and you tell them it is cancer you have to be prepared for particular reactions; a kind of drawing back, embarrassment, almost as if they had shamed you by exposure. "Oh, I'm sorry" is followed by a hasty change of subject and then perhaps a flimsy excuse about an urgent errand that permits departure.

"Come too close and you will be contaminated. I am unclean." Cancer is the leprosy of our time. I do sometimes feel unclean. I never felt that way before during other illness. Perhaps it is the very nature of the disease and the bodily symptoms. Even now, sometimes I really hate those ugly cancerous growths. But the dread of "contamination" is out of all proportion, and one does not expect this reaction from close friends. I remembered the patients who told me about their friends who avoided them, the excuses for not coming to visit, the fear of "catching it." But I wasn't prepared the first time it happened to me. Someone who for many years had shared our Christmas dinner called to say she would not be able to come this year. The reason seemed unclear. Then came sudden realization and it became all too clear. This happens to other people, not to me, I thought.

Some weeks later, quite unexpectedly, this friend knocked at the door, entered, and sat down as far away from me as possible, by an open window. I recognized and felt her fear. At first we talked of generalities. I then introduced the dreaded topic and found myself trying to reassure her. Eventually she got up to go, hurried along the hall, and then stopped and turned and with tear-filled eyes flung her arms around me, kissed me, and was gone. I have never forgotten that incident because of the courage she summoned up to come and because of her final gesture, overcoming fear.

5
Peace and Calm

IN THE beginning the diagnosis of cancer did not portend death to me. I know many women who have had breast cancer, survived, and are well many years later. I was busy coping with the disease and treatments and trying to carry on with my work with the bereaved families. I had grown used to illness interrupting my life and this was just another one, at first. But then came evidence that the disease was spreading. Realization of the outcome came gradually as each effort to halt its progress was unsuccessful.

One day the surgeon was suddenly too busy to return my phone calls. Previously, appointments had been made easily and consultations arranged quickly. Now all this changed. I began to remember that a surgeon's time is precious and must be reserved for patients for whom treatment may bring cure. I knew then that I had become one of the failures. Perhaps too my surgeon had personal difficulty in confronting death or his dying patients. I remembered the patients and families who had spoken of being abandoned by their doctors and the terrible feelings of helplessness and hopelessness that ensued. I understood. I was fortunate, however, and still am, in that I had never lacked medical help and support. Many times physician friends have come to bring relief and help by day or night and I always know that someone will come if I ask.

The cancer continued to spread.

People began to ask me what I felt about suicide. Did I not now sometimes consider such a possibility? At first I was surprised by the question. I thought that the real pain of a terminal illness was that it causes life to end too soon. The question seemed to suggest that it was life that one might want to escape from, not death. Still, for me, life, though painful and difficult sometimes, had never seemed intolerable and what remaine of it became infinitely more precious when I knew that it m ght end soon.

Looking back now I realize that there could be many reasons why terminally ill people do sometimes end their own lives. At the beginning there are so many fears, and so many unknowns lie ahead. Fear may be the greatest enemy; fear of unrelieved pain and suffering, fear of losing control, fear of becoming a burden, physically, emotionally, or financially, to those one loves.

Sometimes these things do happen and the burdens seem too great. In some places, where people have to pay their own medical expenses, they see their financial resources being completely drained. They realize that an accumulation of debts will be the only financial legacy they will be able to leave behind for those they love and had expected to support.

Thinking about these things, I realize how fortunate I have been. Through my work I knew from the beginning that in most cases it is now possible to control the pain and other symptoms that could make life seem intolerable. Medicare and private insurance take care of the medical bills. Loving friends and family continue to support and care for me. So far the burdens have not been too great and I have tried to ensure that they will not be. For me, there are not too many fears left.

I have always felt that I can and should fight back against the disease with every resource that is available. This I continue to do. But at the same time I know that it is possible to accept whatever course it takes.

I am particularly fortunate in that I still have the opportunity to use my own experiences to help others a little, even when I have to remain in bed. I listen to and think about other people's problems, which often are much greater than my own. Mine do not seem so very terrible; I can still forget

46

about them sometimes.

Even so, inevitably spells of depression occur that have to be lived through, times of loneliness, and many painful losses along the way. There are times when one's whole perspective on life seems to get distorted and the task of coping becomes very difficult. But I know that these times do pass. I have to remind myself that, although I may be physically diminishing and losing bodily strength, it is still possible to grow spiritually through whatever comes, and that this is what really counts.

I may well be thankful when the time comes and the long struggle is over but I do not think that I shall end life by my own volition. Suicide evades life, not death, and for me life is still a precious gift. The challenge of each day is to make its living worthwhile.

And one never knows what tomorrow will bring. There have been and still are many good things along the way. Life-threatening illness brings gifts as well as sorrows and, paradoxically, one of the most important of the gifts is time, time to come to terms with all kinds of things. One realizes which things in life are important and which are trivial. One can sort out the priorities and perspectives. One learns not to take anyone or anything for granted. Each day becomes important. One also learns that it helps not to take everything too seriously, to look for the lighter side. It's usually there, although sometimes it gets hidden a bit. It helps not to descend into the doom and the gloom.

Appreciation comes for all kinds of things that previously have been taken for granted. I think particularly of an experience I had soon after the word *terminal* was being used to describe my illness.

During an unexpected last fierce snow storm that spring I suddenly felt an overwhelming urge to go out and feel and savour it to the full. I rushed out and stood looking up as the snowflakes drifted down around me. As I stood there I wondered, "Will this be the last time?" This was not a sad experience; it was a joy. I saw those snowflakes in a way that I had never really seen before. I felt myself absorbing some of their intrinsic beauty, to be remembered especially during times of pain or stress. That memory is still there, providing a kind of strength. If I hadn't had cancer and if I hadn't known that I was going to die I doubt if I would have given the day a second thought. There have been, and still are, many similar experiences. These are the gifts of life-threatening illness. One never knows when the next one will appear.

The experience of having worked among people who are dying can be of great help when one is confronted with one's own death. I have been with people as they died; I have watched and seen. It is true that sometimes the experiences were painful, but I know that death can be gentle and a time of peace.

I remember very specially the death of one lady in the hospital ward. Separated from her husband, she had lived alone with her two young daughters for several years. They were very close. The mother had seemed anxious and agitated as she became sicker and weaker. On the last night of her life the girls came into the ward carrying a guitar, accompanied by a few of their teen-aged friends. People in the ward raised their eyebrows because everybody knew that the mother was very close to death. No other relatives were present. The girls entered their mother's room, quietly kissing her and sitting on either side of the bed. No words were spoken. One of them began to play a gentle melody on the guitar, and together, very softly, thay all sang her favourite songs. While they were singing, a look of great peace and calm came over the mother's face and she died.

Being there was one of the most beautiful and moving experiences I've ever had.

6
Pain

As TIME went on I began to think more about my own death. Like so many others I did not really fear death as such but I recognized personal fears about dying, such as experiencing certain symptoms that I knew to be very unpleasant. I wouldn't like to choke to death, nor would I like to be in such great pain that I would lose self-control. But I was fortunate in that I had already seen that even the most distressing problems can be alleviated by a caring staff.

As my disease advanced, pain did become increasingly the main problem. Its control has been one of the most important facets of the care I have received, the single thing for which I am the most grateful.

The disease spread and the pain increased but I was reluctant to accept strong medication because I was afraid that I would become drowsy, unable to think clearly, unable to function. Because it seemed important to continue to function normally for as long as possible, I postponed taking the medication for a long time and suffered considerable distress in the process. A bottle of Brompton Mixture (containing ten milligrams of morphine per dose) stood on my bedside table untouched for nearly a month while I struggled to cope and to resist the temptation.

Finally I realized that I was reaching a point where I wasn't really able to function at all. All I could think about was the pain — chronic, excruciating pain. It never went away, never allowed a night's sleep. It was always there. I was engulfed by it and felt as if I were trapped in a kind of shell, curled up with the tension of it all. Desperately, I hung on to self-control, trying not to scream as something gnawed at my bones. It was impossible to think of anything or anyone else. At last I realized that not only was I in great distress but that the people who cared were also greatly upset.

C.S. Lewis, who witnessed his wife's pain as she was dying of cancer, compared it with his own torment and suffering during bereavement. "What is grief compared with physical pain?" he asked. "Whatever fools may say, the body can suffer twenty times more than the mind. The mind has always some power of evasion. At worst the unbearable thoughts only come back and back but the physical pain can be absolutely continuous. Thought is never static — pain often is."[7] I think he is right.

The day arrived when I accepted my first dose of the Brompton Mixture. Drowsiness overcame me just as I had feared and had been predicted, but the pain faded away. For three days I slept and wakened, aware of very little. Drugged sleeping, however, changed to dozing and gradually even the drowsiness left. I was alert and the pain had gone.

I find it impossible to describe the relief, the gratitude, that I felt. As if by magic the pain had left and with it the fear that it would return. I relaxed. My mind felt clear and my energy was restored. I came out of my shell and into the world again, interacting with other people and thinking about and planning how I could get back to helping.

So it has gone on. The cancer is widespread and the morphine dose has gradually increased. But although I now require nearly 100 milligrams of morphine every four hours (it has been so for more than a year), I believe that my mind remains reasonably clear. I tire easily and need to sleep more, but there is also more disease in my body. Sometimes there is some pain. But I can adjust the dose to bring complete relief if I want, which I do when I am ready to sleep, or I lower it a little when I want to be especially alert, to write.

I know how fortunate I am. Occasionally I reread the lines a very courageous English lady (whose family I know well) wrote in her published diary shortly before she died of cancer ten years ago, and I realize how it might have been for me.

"Now an intolerable longing for death. Unimaginable pain and purgatory. Mental and physical agony. How long can I continue with it? All hope is gone, only the longing for death remains. I can't take my own life without hurting so many others but sometimes I wonder how long it will be before this is the only endurable solution to such indescribable agony. Why should one be so bitterly tested? The end need not always be so savage."[8]

A highly intelligent, wealthy woman, she had had every advantage and luxury in life. In the 1960s, however, Brompton Mixture did not exist. The progress of her disease had been very similar to my own. But for me the agony is gone. I have been given the opportunity to really live each day that is left. None must be wasted.

Last winter we had a serious fire in our apartment building. Smoke seeped in through the front door and billowed up from the floor. In a very few minutes the whole place was filled with it. Exit from the front of the building was obviously impossible. We hurried to the kitchen door, Louise clutching our little dog and helping me along.

Suddenly I turned and hurried back into the smoke of my bedroom. Louise called to me to come — there was no time — nothing could be saved but ourselves. "Never mind the jewelry, the money, the passports, the bonds, whatever it is you are trying to get."

I came back choking and gasping and collapsed at the door. I was helped out, still clutching the one thing that I had saved: my precious bottle of Brompton Mixture! Did I say that in dying one learns to set priorities?

7
Experiment

ONE DAY the Brompton Mixture was brought by the nurse as usual. No comment was made. Later, when I took it out of the paper bag I saw it was a different colour. I removed the cap and noticed a different smell; no longer did it have the aroma of a cough mixture. I tasted it and that was different too — orange flavour, sickly sweet. Obviously this was not the usual mixture. I read the label. The contents were listed exactly as before. I didn't believe it. Perhaps there had been some mistake and I had received another patient's bottle, someone who could not tolerate the chloroform water. Although I didn't like this new flavour, it was a trivial matter and I decided not to mention it but just to wait until the next batch arrived.

When the next bottle arrived, no remarks were made about it. I unwrapped it. The contents were listed exactly as always, but again I knew that such was not the case. I wondered whether I was supposed to pretend that I did not see, smell, or taste any difference. What was going on? Several physician friends mentioned in turn that they knew experiments were being made with the Brompton Mixture. They asked if I was being included. (Hospital physicians had been asked to give notification if they did not wish their patients to be involved.)

Still no one said a word and neither did I. I remembered patients and families telling me, "They experiment with drugs on the dying cancer patients, you know. We have no say; they never tell us what they do." I had always denied that this could happen and suggested that the only experiments might be to find what drugs suited individual needs and that patients would be told about it. Now I was not so sure. I waited with interest and some chagrin to see what would happen next.

One day the telephone rang. A young man introduced himself by name and hospital affiliation and said that he would read a list of adjectives and I should tell him which best described my pain at that moment. No further explanation was offered. I complied.

A few days later came a repeat of the phone call. I tried to explain that my answer could not have much meaning if it was being related to the effectiveness of the Brompton Mixture because I had had chemotherapy and had vomited all the mixture that day. I was being given morphine injections instead. He told me he did not require that information; I was just to give the adjective appropriate to my pain.

A few days later, after two unsuccessful attempts at nerve blocks, my discomfort was severe. During the phone call I attempted to explain and was cut short again. I realized that the young man had orders that were plain and clear: only one simple answer was to be given. No details or explanations were to be recorded.

Moreover, this was a difficult time for me. Metastases were being diagnosed and new symptoms were appearing. I felt that I really needed the security of the pain-controlling drugs that I knew so well, that they were the one thing that I could count on. I realized that the cocaine was probably absent and I was wondering if I was feeling edgy and nervous because of this or because I no longer felt secure. The label lied, and I began to feel that so did those I had trusted. Did they really think that I didn't notice any difference? As for the phone calls, surely anyone would wonder why this sudden interest had arisen.

Eventually I made it known that I realized the Brompton Mixture had changed. I explained that I was feeling upset by it and that my inclusion in these experiments at that particular time could not really provide useful information.

The message was relayed but the experiments continued as before. No reply or explanation was offered. I am a patient. I meekly answered each call, volunteering nothing that was not directly asked.

One day the mixture sprouted a fungus type of mold. Was the preserving alcohol removed? No, the label still says ethyl alcohol 94 percent, 2.5 milliliters per 20 milliliter-dose, cocaine 10 milligrams (I know that that is not so), chloroform water added to make up the 20 milliliters per dose (it simply isn't there). What's left unchanged — the morphine content? Will that be the next to go?

One day when I was late for a hospital appointment, a taxi waiting at the door, the phone rang. I started to explain that the time was not convenient and asked to be called back or I would call back later. I was told, "This will only take three minutes and it has to be now." I was asked to give the adjective that was appropriate to my pain and also to answer whether I felt "oriented as to time, place, and space?" If I hadn't laughed I think I would have cried.

Another day, a procedure had been very difficult. The question came. The answer was "excruciating." What was the reply? "Thank-you and good-bye." I thought, "Special care for the dying? Is this what it's become?" The warmth and gratitude were turning to anger, frustration, and helplessness. Worst of all, where was that all-important trust now? This was an essential experiment? Surely there must be some other way. Perhaps I was overreacting because such a short time ago these people were my colleagues and my friends. I should not expect special privileges.

Other physician friends knew of my distress and urged me to let them prescribe the Brompton Mixure as before, arguing that the changes and uncertainty were detrimental and an added burden at a difficult time of fast-spreading metastases. Knowing that I could always change my mind, I decided to continue and experience the whole experiment as all the others must who lacked my opportunity. But I would keep a record of events and my reactions; maybe someday someone would care to know just how a patient felt.

I knew that my reactions had been very much influenced by personal circumstances. I decided to make enquiries about some of the other patients who had been involved. I discovered that several home-care patients had become similarly anxious and alarmed when they had noticed changes, but they had not liked to complain.

One day some months later, by chance I had the opportunity of meeting the young medical student who had been involved. I told him that I was interested to know how he felt about having to reply to people in excruciating pain in such an unconcerned way. He replied, "I hated it. There were many nights when I couldn't sleep while I was having to do that." I smiled and told him that I felt better about him. I asked but never did find out the results of the experiments. I still hope there may be a publication one can read at some point. One thing I know is that six months later the Brompton Mixture was changed, I suppose for all the patients. The chloroform water was replaced by the orange syrup. The cocaine was removed and the alcohol reduced by 50 percent. I know this because one day there was a different list of contents on the bottle.

8
A Member of a
Helping Team Is Dying

The wind of heaven blows
The anchor desperately clutches the mud,
And my boat is beating its breast against the chain.[9]

WHEN WORD spread that I had cancer I received much kindness, attention, and support from every member of the hospital ward staff. I was sustained and uplifted by it. But above all, I felt tremendous gratitude for the way in which they helped and encouraged me to continue to participate in the work. For a long time I still felt like one of the team, which was tremendously important to me.

At times I sensed fear in some faces. I realized that when one of the care-givers "succumbs" it's hitting close to home. (It can't be denied; we could be next.) But I tried to let them see that it really wasn't so very terrible. Life still held much that was good.

My studies were read with enthusiasm and appreciation. I was invited to resume attendance at bereavement meetings. Someone was always ready to meet me with a wheelchair at the hospital entrance and often someone would drive me home afterward.

I was told that new staff appointments would preclude further work on the wards, which, although I understood, was a disappointment. This was where I had always felt most able to help in the past, and now I felt that I had more to offer. I believed that new insight and understanding had come with my own cancer and I wished I could use it. But perhaps it would have been too soon.

My involvement in bereavement work had grown out of my time of personal incapacity. It was absorbing and fascinating, so I was glad to be able to continue to be involved in it. I felt happy and fully occupied, even when metastases became evident and symptoms a problem. I was able to keep busy working at home on my own. I planned new studies, making the telephone calls and writing and typing records and results. One day a tiny nurse, who had noticed my physical difficulties in typing, appeared at the door lugging a heavy electric typewriter she had collected for me. The hospital ward paid for its hire for many months so that I could more easily continue with my work.

I was able to attend the hospital meetings, which seemed important for keeping up to date with developments. But I was careful not to intrude or offer suggestions unless specifically asked. I contributed very little overtly when I attended. Perhaps I was too cautious. I knew that I was becoming more and more of an onlooker. I also knew that for many my role was changing — a colleague was becoming a patient and sometimes, I felt, an embarrassment. I think this occurred gradually as my disease spread and people began to realize that it was now appropriate to regard me as "dying."

So much is written in the literature of thanatology about how people do not change fundamentally when they are dying and that they cope with this crisis in the way that they have coped with the other crises in their lives. Yet, just like "cancer," the label of "dying" brings about a strong reaction, perhaps not so much in very personal relationships, but certainly with fellow workers, even in a caring staff of experts. It is as if one has changed. One feels that one is set apart. One notices an alteration in what is felt to be the comfortable distance between others and oneself; a kind of displacement occurs. There is no longer the same free interaction. A kind of barrier seems to have been set up.

The staff became more careful about what they said. Discussion of a patient whose disease resembled my own became an embarrassment if I was present. Someone would begin to talk as usual and then trail off. I realized I was becoming an impairment to their work. There are helpers and

64

there are patients; one apparently cannot be both. I felt in a kind of no-man's land for a while, and then I crossed the line. I understood, but the experience was frustrating. It came at a time when, having experienced first-hand so many of the feelings and symptoms that patients described, I felt that I had more to offer now, not less. Moreover, I was beginning to feel a small sense of urgency. The knowledge that there might not be very much time gave me a strong desire not to waste what I had. It was hard to be so close and yet not allowed to act.

When someone has been bereaved it is generally suggested that he or she should wait a year before attempting to help others in similar circumstances. I have always thought that this was sound advice, as recovery from one's own grief is necessary before one can function efficiently in this capacity.

But you can't wait until you have actually died before you help the dying. There is no coming back. I think standards have to be a little different.

If one has never been seriously ill, and if the diagnosis of cancer is recent, one may still be enmeshed in the turbulent feelings that will inevitably arise and one may not be completely objective. But if one has already lived through many years of life-threatening illnesses, as I have, and if the cancer has been present for several years, I think there is reason to consider that useful contribution might still be possible.

It is often said that the longer the illness, the more depressed one is likely to become. I have not found this to be so in my own life. I do have my ups and downs but I feel that time has brought strengthening and new understanding. One seems to develop a particular kind of sensitivity: one can see and recognize in others the unspoken fears and the pain that one has known.

To be pushed aside into a state of psychological and sociological death before one's body dies seems such a waste if one has a useful contribution to make. Of course, the value of the contribution and not one's personal satisfactions has to be the deciding factor.

Thus I found myself frustrated. I was trying too hard, asking to help and being refused. All kinds of thoughts crossed my mind. I wondered whether they were protecting me, feeling that I was making it all harder for myself knowing that if I had to give up trying to help I could and would die more easily and quickly. I knew they cared very deeply about me. "Perhaps," I thought, "I should have more confidence in their judgment." Yet I also wondered whether they were protecting themselves from a peculiar kind of self-reproach that I think my presence sometimes brings or the hurt they fear if I stay too close. "They have to remain strong to function," I reminded myself. "There are so many to be helped. This must be the priority." But in the back of my mind was still the sense of urgency — "There may not be much more time. I cannot waste it!"

I remember receiving a letter from Father Benedict Vanier. Often I have been guided and uplifted by the gentle wisdom of his letters. I had spoken to him of my personal dilemma at this point. That day he wrote to me about the interaction of "just being" and "being of service." "Never let the desire to help become anxious or compulsive," he advised. "Let it be gentle, abandoned, relaxed. Let it be surrounded with a complete gift in the relative incapacity, and happy with a very limited 'output.' But in its gentleness, gift, serenity, it will be witness to Him and bring to others your presence and help — however small." I have read those words many times to remind myself of their wisdom.

One day soon after this, a nurse asked me if I would be willing to go and talk with a patient who was very afraid of dying. She thought that perhaps I could help. I said that I would be glad to try if there was no objection from other staff members.

9
Melanie

The Bird of Time has but a little way
To fly — and Lo! the Bird is on the Wing.[10]

I WAS TOLD that Melanie was a young married woman who had never been sick before. Suddenly diagnosis was made of advanced lung cancer. She was very upset and was having great difficulty in accepting the disease and her own impending death.

When I went to see her I was met at the hospital entrance by the kind friend who had so many times taken me in the wheelchair to and from the ward. She deposited me at the door of Melanie's room and left.

I knocked and entered and saw an attractive young woman sitting up in bed, talking to a medical student. Melanie was expecting me. She turned eagerly to greet me and then introduced me by name to the student, adding, "She used to work here. She used to do social work. But now she is just like me. She's dying too."

For a moment I was taken aback. I know now that I had entered that room as I had done so many times in the past, anticipating the comfortable distance that would allow me to use the skills of my trade, giving me time to assess and learn her needs, her desire for closeness and for sharing. Immediately, however, I had been given the message — not this time! Professional skills are not what she wants from me. She asked me to come for just one reason: "she is dying too."

I had been fortunate in having had close and caring friends who had understood and listened patiently to all the things I had needed to say and discuss. I didn't feel a need to share now, and certainly not with a stranger. But I knew then that if I was really going to help I had to share, to let myself be open and exposed.

At first it was hard to do this; I felt vulnerable. Melanie asked many questions. "How do you cope? When you wake up in the morning can you really believe that it's true? How do you get through the day? Have you any idea what it will really be like to die?"

I realized how intensely lonely she felt in her present situation and I wanted very much to help her. She told me about trying to put up a good front, pretending that everything was all right, but she was terrified and angry too. She was young and had never been ill before. This couldn't be true. Why should it happen to her? She had always been the strong one. She couldn't die!

During the following weeks and months we had many long talks in her hospital room, and on other occasions she would telephone me at home when she wanted to talk. She seemed to relate very freely to me and we discussed all kinds of things — her thoughts and feelings, the way the disease was progressing in both of us, the things that were happening in her life. Some matters were personal and confidential and others were not so private. She was very much afraid of the actual experience of dying, so I told her about some of the times I had been present when people died. I was able to tell her how I had seen distressing symptoms controlled and eased by the special caring staff on her ward. I told her too of the times I had been very close to death, explaining that they were different from the present moment as we sat there talking. I had become so tired and weak that even to breathe was an effort. Death had not seemed terrible at all. I suggested that perhaps it would be this way for us both in the end.

I told her too that with time I had become more used to the prospect of death and that it did not disturb me so much anymore. But the present was much more precious now, and it seemed important to make the most of each day.

One day she told me about a priest who had come to see her and who had suggested that if she were to offer the rest of her life to some new service for God and if she would give all her money to charity God might heal her. Later, when she had found her own way back to faith, she was able to laugh at this bargaining with God.

She talked of the pressures being put upon her to make her will and her reluctance to do so, interpreted by many as an unwillingness to take the step that would indicate that she really knew that she was going to die. As she talked, it quickly became obvious that the reason for her reluctance was something else. She had decided that the weak person who loved her but had let her down so many times should not have the inheritance. This person would never use it wisely. Common sense dictated that it should go elsewhere. Our conversation, however, made her realize that she really wanted to forgive, and here, in this last giving, was the opportunity to express her love, confidence, and hope. Foolish? Maybe. But the will was written in a matter of minutes and her relief was great.

As she grew sicker and weaker, occasionally a notice was posted on her door saying that she wanted no visitors but me. I still wondered a little sometimes. I knew she felt very close to me and that she could talk easily and freely without restraint, but I also knew that there were others, members of the staff who had come very close to her too. Then one day she said, "People are so kind to me; they have all been kind and good to me. I feel especially close to some. But with you there is one big difference and in a way it goes beyond the fact that we both have cancer and are dying. You see, they are well. I find myself getting to know and getting very fond of them but I don't want to get too close — I'm going to have to leave them all behind. With you I can get close and share as we talk. It's as if we are going on a kind of journey together. We sort of plan together. I won't have to leave you behind."

Her words brought new meaning. I even felt that they gave me some small glimpse of the "why" of my own illness.

Melanie died quietly and peacefully one night soon afterwards. I was sad and I missed her, but the whole experience had been a kind of gift.

I was filled with hope that I might be asked to go back some other time if need arose. I knew that I had found the capacity to reach out to another person, to drop the barriers and relax, to really help.

A week after Melanie's death there was a staff meeting, the subject of which was Melanie's illness and death. Someone told me about it later. I should have liked to have been there. I think perhaps the staff had thought it might have been upsetting for me to attend. I know some felt that I should not have been asked to visit Melanie. They knew that my physical condition was rapidly deteriorating. Yet I think I was less upset by her death than many of them. In many ways I felt strengthened by the experience. It had been a very special privilege to share that little fragment of Melanie's journey.

But this was to be the last time I was asked to go back to the hospital ward.

Tired
And lonely
So tired
The heart aches.
Meltwater trickles
Down the rocks,
The fingers are numb,
The knees tremble.
It is now,
Now, that you must not give in.

* * *

Weep
If you can,
But do not complain.
The way chose you —
And you must be thankful.[11]

72

10
Hurt and Healing

My clouds, sorrowing in the dark,
forget that they themselves
have hidden the sun.[12]

SHORTLY AFTER Melanie died I realized that I was no longer being invited to meetings or to hear visiting guest speakers or to attend social gatherings. Certain staff members had visited me regularly. This had started at the time of their first involvement in bereavement follow-up, when they wanted to talk of their experiences, to discuss and plan how best to help the families and how to cope with their own personal reactions. They had continued to come or telephone, and some now talked of more personal matters. Since I was at this point out of the hospital setting and yet aware of the general situation and the problems and stresses, these people seemed to find it helpful to come and talk. In particular, there was someone who cared very deeply about the patients and tended to be devastated by their deaths. We had begun to talk a lot about this problem, the possible reasons for it, and this person's own personal life.

But then warning was given that I was going to die and that if people allowed themselves to get too close they would be hurt. The "vulnerable" person specifically was forbidden to come to see me. I wondered, did no one realize that I was well aware of the risks and the weaknesses and the vulnerability but that I might just conceivably be able to help, not harm? Again, my big regret was the lack of direct communication. I think we could all have benefited from open discussion. I realize that when one is alone with time to spare there is a tendency to blow things up out of proportion, and perhaps they were right. Yet I felt a strong inner conflict. I could not jeopardize anybody or the work. I would not support defiance of the decision, as those who were involved suggested, but I would not refuse to help anyone who asked. The telephone was my compromise.

A staff member came to see me and said, "You know, the whole trouble with you is that you haven't followed the rules. People were prepared to support and help you for a certain length of time. But you didn't die when you were supposed to. They didn't expect you to go on for so long. They don't know how to cope with you now.

"If you had only stayed in bed, stopped trying to help and be a part of the service, you might have died a year ago. Everyone would have looked after you. You would have had a splendid funeral — who knows, they might even have erected a stained-glass window to your memory!

"Now you make people uncomfortable. You still insist on doing your own thing and because you succeed some even see you as a rival and a threat. You know, you really blew it!" These were strong words, laughingly said with tongue-in-cheek, but I recognized a lot of truth in them.

I recognized it again a short time ago when a visitor looked at me and said, "So you're still fighting then?" I smiled. What was there to say? I suppressed the chuckle that came to the surface as I realized how close I had come to apologizing and making excuses for still being alive.

I know now that I expected too much when I assumed that working relationships could continue as before, for as long as physical strength permitted.

For a while I was frequently told, "You are an example and inspiration to us all." I felt myself being placed on a kind of pedestal. But pedestals are for statues, impossible positions for living human beings to hold. I am no statue, no saint, and very human. I am not sure when I fell off my particular pedestal but I know that for some I did. I'm still up there for others but theirs is a distant view.

I think perhaps I became less "saintly" after some people noticed I was hurt when certain incidents occurred. I realize now that they were probably a series of misunderstandings. My studies were included in a published volume without mention of the author. The day of an international symposium I watched as one of my studies was presented. Slides had been made of my diagrams and graphs, and I saw them all up there on the screen and heard the details of my work. I should have been proud, but I was deeply hurt. No one had even told me that it was to be used, let alone asked permission to do so. My name was never mentioned.

I remember going home, exhausted and spent, and collapsing into bed and crying. I forgot for a time the pleasure I had had in doing the work, that I had offered it freely in the hope that it might be helpful, and that this was all that really mattered.

I was lying in my bed of self-pity when the telephone rang and a voice at the other end said, "This is Elisabeth. We're having a little get-together. Please come." I replied, "I'd love to come and see you but I'm in bed and very, very tired — really exhausted. I just don't think that I can make it." "Do come," she responded, "even if only for a few minutes. We will fill you with so much love we'll take away all the tiredness." I couldn't resist. Somehow I dressed and went and it was as she said. I understood and experienced first-hand the strength of the warmth and love that Dr. Elisabeth Kübler-Ross has brought to so many of her dying patients and friends. I don't know how or if she had sensed or understood my hurt that night when she telephoned, and although I have seen her many times since then I have never told her the story, but I know and remember what she did for me.

11
Changing Relationships

The tapestry of life's ties is woven
With the threads of life's ties ever joining and breaking.[13]

A SHORT TIME after the party, a physician I had met that night came to visit me. We talked for a long time of many things. When he got up to leave, he said, "You know, when I asked about coming to see you I was told that you are going through a stage of anger just now, but I have never met anyone who seems so tranquil and filled with peace."

After he left, I thought about what he had said. I knew that friends had protested and made known my hurt about my studies. But it seemed to me that the real problem was that the label of "dying" had intervened again. I realized how easy it is to interpret each action and reaction as a direct consequence of being in the process of dying. If each time one is angry it is called part of the "normal" state of dying, it doesn't really have to be dealt with. It doesn't matter whether the anger is justified. It can be labelled "displaced." When one is very ill it can be said that one overreacts to many things. (One can also become frustrated and angry at times. That person "who does not change basically because he is dying" feels helpless and impotent.)

I now know that I was being protected from the unpleasantness of confrontations and disagreements. But I didn't see it that way. I thought perhaps people were protecting themselves, not me. What I could not see, of course, was that all those people, who really cared greatly, were watching as I grew physically more and more weak and ill. Being so eager to go on helping, I must have made the decision very hard for them. The time had come when they felt that I should be asked to do no more. I had to accept that I could no longer be a part of the hospital service.

Mine was a difficult bereavement. I struggled through a personal "Slough of Despond" as I realized that the active part of my working life was ended.

I have felt a great reluctance to write about this. I have received and I continue to receive a great deal of genuine love, care, and kindness from all these people. It seems ungrateful to write so much about what are such minor and trivial matters. This is not a catharsis; that came long ago. Several things have happened, however, that make me feel that I should make known some of the difficulties and problems I have experienced as a member of a helping team.

An eminent psychiatrist who is also a friend told me of problems encountered when a member of a team in another hospital died of cancer. He told me that the staff felt that they had somehow failed to help this one person whom they had most wanted to support. He asked me to write about my own experiences. It seems to me unlikely that any of my story will be useful. I know, though, that many others are and will be involved as helpers who will tread similar paths in the future. Several incidents have made me realize that we have much in common.

Recently, during a seminar on terminal care, this same psychiatrist mentioned my studies in his presentation and quoted from my writings. (He not only mentioned me by name but introduced me to the participants!) Afterward, a young woman came up to me and said, "I am Claudia Behrendt. I am a nurse and I look after very sick children. I have leukemia, and since my own diagnosis I have had a most difficult and frustrating time. I feel now that I can understand my patients better and help them more than I could before but I'm constantly frustrated. The staff's whole attitude has changed: they protect me; they don't give me a chance anymore. When I listened today and heard about your work and the way you have carried on with it I wanted to have an opportunity to talk to you, to find out how it is that you have managed to find the way to do it. I want to carry on for as long as I am able but it doesn't seem possible. How do you do it?"

Conversation was interrupted, but we have corresponded since. Claudia sent me some of the poems she had written and hopes to have published and some extracts from her diary. At the time of her first remission she wrote, "I can remember trying to put myself in my patient's place — guessing what he was thinking, what he expected me to say. I really thought I understood until I was diagnosed as having acute myoblastic leukemia. I thought I had achieved understanding and empathy with dying patients and families. Now I find that some of the clichés I once used to console patients are the same ones that manage to upset me the most. I have learned so much and after a long recovery I am facing the return to the job I love."[14]

She talked of her own needs when she wrote, "What I am really stiving for now is to get things back to what they were before. They will never be exactly the same — I realize this but I need to have things as normal and active as possible to give me the strength to handle the constant reminders and side effects of the chemotherapy and illness."

Shortly after this, she wrote of the frustrations and disappointments: "Most of the time I feel branded. I feel I should apologize for dying because it makes others feel uncomfortable and therefore I feel uncomfortable. I think I try always to be extra cheerful and laughing so I don't put anyone on the spot!"

Claudia gave me permission to use her notes with my own. We hope that they may help in some small way to further understanding.

12
Youth and Death

You whisper about my youth but when one is dying
is he really so young anymore?"[15]

I OFTEN THINK about Claudia and about how it must be to face death at her age. I think too of those poignant lines that open this chapter, written in 1970 by another young nurse. My mind goes back to a time some thirty years ago when, as a young girl, I too lay close to death. It was the middle of the night, an emergency admission by ambulance to the women's ward of a hospital in England. Curtains were quickly drawn around the bed. Recollections of the night are hazy: total exhaustion; excruciating pain that seemed unending; the visit of the surgeon in the small hours of the morning; a hurried, gentle examination; words whose only reassurance offered some relief from the horrible pain. Then came injections and the pain ebbed for a time of merciful, drugged sleep.

Very early in the morning, a trolley rattling on its way stopped briefly outside my curtained cubicle. Ambulatory patients were bringing the traditional, all-important, early morning cup of tea to the bedridden. I clearly heard the whispering voices. "Did you see her when they brought her in last night, pale as a ghost, so sick and weak; she looked so young. They say she is going to die. Fair breaks your heart. She can't be more than fourteen years old. A dreadful thing to die so young! I couldn't sleep all night for thinking about her. She's just a child!" Cups rattled and on they went.

I remember very clearly how surprised I was by what they had said. It seemed so strange. What difference did it make that I was young — ten years or a hundred years (in fact seventeen)? Pain, relentless and continuing, is not kinder to the young, nor is the lack of sleep, nor the long time of sickness and weariness. How merciful would be the sleep that would end it all. There was no bitterness. I do not even remember fear: only a sense of aloneness. Can it be that, in dying, we are old beyond our years?

Perhaps this was a particular time in the stages of life, a kind of threshold: the time before I fell in love; the time before I read about Octavia Hill and planned single-handedly to carry on her torch and eradicate the slums of London. It was also during the war, so death was familiar and close to us all.

In those wartime days, idealism was channelled into patriotic zeal. The many young men who faced death and those who died in battle became the heroes and the martyrs to the cause of freedom. Swept along on the emotional tides of glory, honour, and patriotism, even the survivors seemed to accept the necessity of the sacrifice as some comfort in their grief. But the soldiers' was a different kind of dying.

Death in battle was often quick, with little time for preparation. Terminal illness brings another kind of battle, which may be long and frustrating but may also give way to final acceptance. Youth looks to the future with strong hopes, ideals, ambitions, and plans. To be cut down in the prime can be excruciatingly painful. The young adult who is dying may experience more intense anger and frustration than a person who dies at any other time of life. Each person responds in his or her own unique way.

For me, it is the middle years of life. Now there is love and commitment. Relationships have been established, responsibilities exist. Dreams and hopes have settled into some kind of reality. This is my time of living. This is my time of dying.

No children, you would say, and yet I have many. There are the old ladies, too, who rely on those daily telephone calls to solve the simple problems that worry and confuse tired old minds. I have friends who care, and a little dog who sits patiently with trusting eyes. Eighteen stray cats live in the stable in the country. People still call to share their sorrow and their joys. I try to finish my work.

Perhaps it does not add up to much. But each one means a lot to me. Everyone of us who is dying can make his or her own list. Inexorably we know we must hurt them all. Inevitably we mourn their loss.

Because we know and are aware, whatever our age, ours is the opportunity to love and give for as long as we may, to try to ensure that the memories will be good and precious — joyful, peaceful, and worth the price of the pain.

13
Springs in the Valley

There is a law in life
When one door closes to us
Another one opens.[16]

Doors CLOSE and others open. I mentioned the psychiatrist who gave public recognition of my work. I sometimes wonder if he realized just how much he did for me that day. I have great respect for him as a person, for his knowledge, his judgement, and his honesty. He restored my self-confidence and gave me the incentive to carry on, to write all this, and he made suggestions about further development of my written studies.

Since then I have found that I am able to continue to help a little with some of the patients who have chosen to remain at home until life ends and the families who take care of them. The telephone is my link with people who are lonely or afraid, those who feel the need to share, to talk. I am once more involved, in a small way. I can use the strength of the good days. I am busy and happy.

Life must be lived at a slower and more gentle pace. No longer can I hope to scale mountains! But there is joy and happiness in the simple things that I can still do. I think of the lines of Psalm 104: "He sendeth the springs into the valleys, which run among the hills. . . ." There are indeed many springs in this valley.

A dear friend has taped all my favourite music. The cassettes are stacked along my bedroom walls. (Sometimes they also become a lending library.) They provide endless pleasure, the sounds for every mood, perhaps the greatest gift of all — another kind of listening. The faithful hospital ward friends and helpers still relieve the physical pain and I know that they are always ready to support and help me through whatever crisis may come. Bereaved people with whom I worked at the beginning, mostly now recovered, still telephone occasionally to tell me about recent events in their lives. It is good to share their happier days after all the pain.

I still meet all kinds of different people. I never know who or what tomorrow will bring, who will call or come to visit. One day a visiting physician came to see me. She was a beautiful young woman, full of radiance and charm. She was warm and friendly, and we chatted easily. She talked of her work with dying patients in different hospital settings, remarking, "You know, sometimes I seem to be getting on so well with a patient, achieving a real sense of closeness as we talk, and then suddenly — like today, I was talking to a woman and abruptly and quite inexplicably she stared at me and then stopped talking and turned in her bed with her back to me and told me to go away. She refused to say another word. I wonder, do you have any idea what I could have done to upset her?"

I looked at her and it came to me in a flash. I had never had the particular experience before but, as soon as she had walked in and greeted me, I had looked up at that lovely young face, glowing with health and vitality, and I had suddenly felt old and tired, ugly, sick, and dull. It was but a momentary and fleeting feeling but strong, and I had been surprised at my reaction.

I laughed and told her what I had felt. Such a thing had never crossed her mind and she said that she had never realized that it could happen. Apparently she had had similar experiences on more than one occasion and had spent a long time searching her mind to try and remember what she could have said or done to give offense or raise a barrier.

Another day, another physician came to see me. Again, we had not met before. It was a social call, and we talked of his work with the dying and of how, up until that time, his experience had been mainly with the very old. He asked me how I could accept what was happening to me without anger and resentment. He asked first if I thought I was being punished by a divine power. I told him that I had never thought of illness in that way. It could not be; a tiny baby dies, a little child; punishment for what? (And wicked though I may have been I don't think I have piled up quite enough sins to justify so many ills, if one measures justice by our earthly standards of crime and punishment.)

He said, "Do you believe there is a God?" When I replied, "I do," he continued, "How can you still believe that there is a God who would bring so much pain and suffering into your life? It isn't fair. You are young. How can you believe that there is a God who would treat you so unfairly?"

The thought came to my mind that we are quick to call adversity unfair, but it is never unfair when we receive a special gift, an experience of love or joy. If one stops to think, one realizes that these things far outweigh the hurts. I tried to explain that although the illness does not seem fair to me now, that is one reason why I am so sure that there is a greater meaning than I can see and understand in my present state. While I live I shall not be able to comprehend, "for now we see through a glass, darkly."[17] I think it is a waste of time to worry and wonder about the "whys." It seems to me that faith and trust give strength to carry on and these are what one really needs. It doesn't seem necessary to probe into the past to try to find proof of previous existence any more than to spend time trying to probe the future, to find out through communication with "spirits" what happens when the body dies. Of course I am curious about what is to come. But I can wait. Sometimes I feel it is presumptuous to probe too much. I don't think one should assume that one could even cope with such knowledge in one's present life.

> Let me not grope in vain in the dark
> but keep my mind still in the faith
>   that the day will break
>   and truth will appear
>   in all its simplicity.[18]

When that time comes I shall know and understand. But now, I want to use whatever time is left for living. I remember the words of Father Benedict: "This is a pilgrimage and we have not here a lasting city. We are going somewhere — not alone."

14
Testing Courage

Often the test of courage is not to die but to live.[19]

My ILLNESS has lasted much longer than anyone thought possible, and so have I. I might be tempted to wonder if I could go on living indefinitely were it not for the many acute medical crises that occur with increasing frequency. Each one brings a sharp reminder that the end could come swiftly and at any time.

As time goes by, I do have less need to talk of dying. Although I am aware that this is interpreted by some as a kind of denial, actually I am even more aware of the inevitability and proximity of death as the disease slowly engulfs my body Death has come to the threshold many times. I feel able to look at the familiar presence without discussion and without any real fear now.

It has been a long road and there have been many changes in my life along the way. In the first months, many people came to offer comfort, support, and advice. Friends and colleagues working in the field of thanatology were naturally interested in a fellow worker facing terminal illness. They all rallied to help and observe. Almost overnight I felt like some kind of celebrity. People came and listened to what I had to say as never before, as if my words were suddenly important. I had to remind myself that I hadn't really changed at all. Diagnosis of terminal illness does not, ipso facto, bring startling revelation and insight.

But the constant stream of visitors did change the normal routines of the household, even more than my illness.

It was all too easy to be flattered by the attention and to forget that all those people and the continuous phone calls might not always be welcomed by the other members of my family, who were struggling to cope with the added tasks of a sickroom. (Inevitably, each visit called for one more tray of tea or coffee.) It took a strong outburst to make me realize just how much extra burden and strain was being needlessly added at that time.

"Our whole lives have been altered, not so much by your illness but by all these people who insist on coming to visit. There's no peace anymore, no chance of the quiet evening together. We need and want to live as normally as we can but they don't give us a chance. The doorbell and the phone never stop. And all they really do is to exhaust you. They don't help. They all want to know how you feel about dying and how you are reacting. Why don't they leave us alone? Why don't they let you live? They talk of nothing but cancer and dying. They bring every book. We listen to all those tapes, to every T.V. program, to the films. We eat, sleep, and live to the sounds of cancer. I am sick to death of the whole business!"

I tried to reduce the number of visits, and I succeeded to a certain extent. But I have always had difficulty in turning people away and I still do. When you are lying in bed, everyone knows you are there, and you can't really pretend to be busy. Many kind people assume that they are doing you a favour by visiting. They don't always realize how quickly one becomes exhausted when one is very ill. There have been many occasions when I have tried to reserve time and strength for a special visitor but have been frustrated and exhausted by an insistent unexpected caller.

But time brought changes as the years passed. "Don't give up on me" is a phrase familiar to every student of thanatology. Inevitably, if one takes too long to die, some people do give up. It is not that they cease to care. It just becomes impossible to keep on giving the extra time and energy, to make those special efforts that can be summoned in time of crisis. Some people move away and others grow tired of offering help to a stubbornly independent friend. One comes to realize that relationships that form and are built up on the supposition that you are dying will not necessarily continue if you don't die.

Gradually our lives settled back to a more normal routine. Visits and phone calls become less frequent, and I was particularly glad that I had somehow managed to continue to do a little work. I missed some of the attention, but I had less strength and energy and I had the greater satisfaction of using what remained in small ways of service.

Nearly four years have now passed and I have survived longer than anyone expected. I began to notice a reawakening of interest. Now it is not "How does it feel to die?" but "Why are you still alive?"

One needs a sense of humour and a certain self-reliance to steer a passage through the waves. It would be easy to be swept up by the flattery and attention, only to plunge down into the abyss of loneliness and depression during what seems to be abandonment. The steadfast love and devotion of the few and faith in the ultimate purpose of it all enable me to carry on in a reasonably placid and contented frame of mind.

Talking to some people who have leukemia has brought realization that they go through these cycles many times. Acute phases of the disease bring all kinds of support and rallying friends. But then remissions occur. Paradoxically, these are often the most difficult times. There is a return of strength and energy but, in many cases, no longer work to fill the hours. Idle days at home, friends all working, little hope for the future — this is the time when many feel bitterly lonely, unhappy, and depressed.

There is nothing special about dying. It is the natural conclusion of all our lives. But living in a state of dying for a long times does bring special kinds of experience. Although often in my work I used to hear colleagues argue that you don't have to be poor to understand poverty, there never was any doubt in my mind that it helps. We who live close to death tend to view things from the same angle, and I believe that because of this we can share and help each other.

There are no short cuts to peace and acceptance. But after all these years of grave illness I find that it is sometimes possible to bring small hopes and strength to others by very simple and delicate communication. (I use the word "delicate" because nothing could be less helpful to a person who is hurting or protesting than the introduction, "I'd like you to meet someone who is coping well. Talk to her and see if she can help you to do the same.") It is difficult to explain, but if we talk, people do sense that is is "all right," and if it is all right for me maybe it will be all right for them too. At the very least we can and do speak freely with one another and perhaps assuage some of the feeling of isolation that dying brings to nearly everyone.

Recently I was talking to a lady who had just been given a diagnosis of terminal cancer. She said, "I am surrounded by many caring people — family and friends. I see them all in a kind of circle around me, out there. They are all so busy discussing, interacting. They are trying to reorganize my life: how to cope, how to deal with all the problems, what they will tell me, what they think I should not know, how best to help me, what must be done. I am stuck here in the middle, quite alone. I have to think how to make it easy for them. I have to make my own decisions. I have to come to terms with this thing, and, in the midst of so many people, I never felt so alone in my whole life."

Another woman, Mary, has had leukemia for several years and is now beginning to grow weaker, with shorter and shorter periods of remission. She has a nineteen-year-old daughter who lives at home with her. There are just the two of them. Pamela, a brilliant student, won a rare scholarship for special studies in a distant university. But she was torn. Eager for the opportunity to advance her career, she nevertheless felt that her place was with her mother for what might well be the last months of her life. There was no possibility of postponing the scholarship.

Mary explained, "Pamela says she wants to stay home with me and refuse the scholarship. She is very close to me now but if she stays with me she may come to resent and even hate me for ruining her life. I couldn't bear that. I don't know how much longer I have to live, but this is her chance of a lifetime and I really want her to take it. But if she goes and I die, will she feel terribly guilty for having left me?"

We talked a lot about this. Mary weighed the cost to herself in terms of the inevitable loneliness and the pain, balanced against her joy and pride in her daughter, the hopes that lay in this opportunity for achievement. She knew what she really wanted to do and she made the choice. She was able to be strong in the implementation of the decision, strong enough to outweigh Pamela's doubts and guilt. She made arrangements for someone to come and stay with her so that Pamela would not worry about her being alone, and she firmly silenced the neighbours when they chided Pamela, "How can you be so selfish and so heartless as to leave your mother alone to die?"

There are likely to be many times when Mary will feel weak and sick and very lonely in the days ahead. She knows this better than anyone. But she has great courage and — yes — we do need each other.

15 Listening

Give sorrow words; the grief that does not speak
Whispers the o'er-fraught heart and bids it break.[20]

My WORK with bereaved people has continued for several years now. After all the studies and research I still find that the most important way of helping, at least initially, is just to listen. This is something I can do even when I am lying in bed.

After someone dies, people seem to need and want very much to talk: to talk about the person who has died, the illness, the dying, and the loneliness they then feel. They may be reluctant to share their feelings with their own families for fear of upsetting them or because their reactions are very different and they may not understand. And friends, even close friends, are often found to avoid contact after a death because they are embarrassed and unsure of how to cope with the situation or what to say. They are afraid of provoking tearful outbursts.

I remember one of the first women with whom I talked about the death of her husband. She was very distressed as she described seeing her close friend in the supermarket. The friend, seeing her, turned back down an aisle to avoid contact with her. The woman was very hurt and found it difficult to understand how or why her friend had acted that way.

When people are grieving they often do express all kinds of strong feelings: anger, guilt, despair, helplessness, hopelessness, and self-pity. One has to listen quietly and patiently without judgement, reproach, or criticism. Then people feel that it is all right to talk openly and honestly. They feel that someone understands and cares. They come to realize that crying is normal and nothing of which they should be ashamed. They need simple reassurance and support at this time. Later it may be possible to help and advise with all kinds of practical problems that may arise. Even warnings not to rush into major decisions while they are upset and probably not thinking very clearly can be important and useful.

At the beginning most people cannot imagine how they will ever get over the terrible loss, the anguish, and the loneliness. Eventually, sometimes after many months, the pangs of grief become less intense and frequent. People begin to remember and to talk of some of the good times that were shared, not just the relatively short but painful time of illness and death. One sees the tide beginning to turn and recognizes that recovery has started.

Nowadays my telephone work includes contact with people who are dying and those who are caring for a dying family member, as well as the recently bereaved. I have many times observed that when family members are able to discuss and share in what is happening, they move together towards gradual acceptance of the death, and the last weeks become a very special time of calm and peace. Memories of the period of love and trust and closeness endure and help to support those who are left.

Time is the special gift of opportunity that victims of sudden or unexpected death cannot experience. Time provides opportunity for practical discussion about the future of the survivors as well as the personal needs of the one who is dying. A dying husband can be reassured by knowing that his wife will be better able to cope because he helps her now. This is something he alone can still do when he may otherwise feel helpless and useless.

Each person is unique. Some prefer not to share and some need to deny death to the end. Each of us must tread our own path and personal wishes must always be respected. Reassurance and support can always be offered. Sometimes people become exhausted and so upset that they cannot think clearly. Gentle, tactful suggestions may help them to see needs that are being overlooked or opportunities that are being missed.

Recently I had many conversations with a lady whose husband was spending the last days of his life at home. They were an elderly immigrant couple and, having no relatives and few friends, were very dependent on each other. They had always been reserved and reticent. As her husband grew sicker the wife became increasingly distraught. One morning she telephoned me and said, "My husband is in a kind of coma. He can't speak. I am afraid I am losing him. He just lies there. I have spent the whole night by his bedside crying and begging him not to leave me. I told him I can't live without him. I'm begging him not to go. Everyone is telling me to stop, that I have to let him go, but I can't!"

I asked her if she thought he was suffering but she was sure that he wasn't; he was lying very peacefully. I asked her if she thought he could understand what she was saying, and she said that she was sure that he could, she could tell by his eyes. I said, "Suppose that this might be the last opportunity that you would have to say something to him that he could still understand. Perhaps there is something special that you would want to tell him. Why don't you think about it a little."

The next morning she phoned me early and said, "Do you know what I did? I sat beside him all night and I held his hand and I told him how much I loved him, how good our life together had been, that those thirty years were the most wonderful years of my life and that I would never forget." She added, "You know, if he had been well I could never have talked to him like that; we never did. He'd have wondered what had come over me. But I did it and it was wonderful to be able to tell him."

The lady's husband died that night. Since then we have talked many times and she has wept in her sorrow and loneliness. Every now and again, however, she will suddenly pause and remember, "But, do you know, I said all those special things to him that last night. I don't know how I managed it, but I did. Somehow I do feel really good about that."

During the years that I have continued to work among bereaved people, friends and acquaintances have often asked, "How can you continue to do this work without becoming terribly depressed now that you are so ill yourself?" In fact, the effects have been the exact opposite of what people suppose. As a person who is dying I am, of course, faced with the certain knowledge that I must lose not just one person but everyone and everything that is dear and precious to me. That is one of the very hard things about dying.

Feeling the sadness and knowing that death is coming closer, one also sees that one's family and friends are looking increasingly sad, worried, and anxious. One feels that one is doing something terrible to them and one is helpless to prevent it. Egocentrically, I believed I was completely devastating people's lives and that they would never recover. This was an added burden to dying and it introduced an element of guilt.

When you listen to and work with bereaved people as I have done, and as they talk about their feelings and experiences and you continue to listen at intervals of six months, a year, even longer sometimes, you begin to realize that gradually they do recover. It can be compared with the slow emergence from a long illness. People begin to pick up the pieces, to take up their lives again, perhaps not always where they left off and often saddened a little by the whole experience. One sees that they do not forget the person who has died (of course one is rather glad about that). Yet at the same time one sees that they are able to resume former activities, to start new ones, to form new relationships. Different things begin to happen in their lives. Sometimes one hears people discussing the possibility of remarriage.

One realizes that although people have been through an extremely difficult part of their lives, which has affected them deeply, both emotionally and physically, eventually they can and do come to accept the loss. They recover and are often strengthened in the process. Most have gained in wisdom and understanding from the experience.

Dr. Parkes describes grief as a kind of price we have to pay for having loved someone.[21] If we had not loved and had the joy of the experience we would not have to suffer the pain of loss. But when people begin to be able to remember and talk about the good things and the happy times they shared, one realizes that they can and do come to feel that it was all worthwhile; the love really was worth the price of the pain. This, of course, brings special comfort to me.

16
Hope

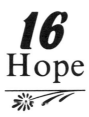

Hope is the thing with feathers
  That perches in the soul,
And sings the tune without the words,
And never stops at all,
And sweetest in the gale is heard.[22]

THERE IS a wondrous order in our universe, and I think that the closer one gets to nature and the simple ways of living the more one can recognize it and accept one's own part in it.

The old friend who bequeathed us her country house bequeathed so much more. She gave us the opportunity for peace and tranquillity, away from the noise and rush of city life. She also enabled us to come very close to birth, life, and death in all their natural ways, to feel a part of it all and to see it from different perspectives.

There are cats in the old stable at the back of the house. Usually they just arrive, abandoned or lost, and settle into the manger, making it their home.

A little while ago I watched the birth of three kittens. The mother cat, a gentle grey-eyed creature, licked her tiny bundles, drank a bowl of milk, and now lies proudly purring close beside them. I don't know where she came from; she was just there when I went in. With her, standing watch, was an enormous ugly tom. The other cats resented his presence but he stood stolidly by until the birth was over, and now he's curled up in a corner of the outer stable, still ready to protect his family, I suppose. As I came back, I passed the little box with the yellow blanket, a special, privileged place. Just a few weeks ago the oldest inhabitant lay sleeping there. She slipped out early one morning and did not come back. Her box is still there, waiting, just in case. But deep down I know she never will return. She knew her time had come. I loved her and I miss her. She was a gentle matriarch, the wisest cat of all.

But the day will come when another unexpected birth occurs, and I know the box with the yellow blanket will be put out to receive some other creature's precious squirming bundles. Birth, life, and death all seem natural here, with all the joys and the pain. The creatures are wild and beautiful, cruel and tender.

Sometimes raccoons or skunks will wander into the stable in the quiet of night. One looks in and sees them sitting placidly beside the cats sharing the leftover supper in the bowls.

Outside there is life too numerous to describe. I can see now from where I sit the hummingbirds and the butterflies hovering over the flowers in my garden and the leaves so green on the magnificent trees. They will all come and go in their seasons — creatures, flowers, plants, and leaves. Some wither and die too soon. But all form the rich compost to provide nourishment for another spring's growth. The continuing cycle becomes a kind of hope. In this place I feel new strength; everything is purified and made simple.

Hope does not die. For each of us, however, it changes a little from time to time.

Last winter I wrote about what it was for me then, saying, "I cannot hope now that my disease will magically disappear." At the beginning of the illness I did hope that it would not spread. But it did. Now, hope is something different. Hope for me means that maybe I'll get to the country to see my garden again next spring and that I'll see the flowers in bloom.

Hope is something that, last autumn, made me work in my garden and plant the bulbs that will come up in the spring, despite people looking at me and saying, "Oh, you're too tired, you're too sick. You shouldn't be trying to do that." What they were thinking but not saying was, "You know you are not going to be alive to see them. Why are you doing it?"

The answer is simple. "I love my garden and I love the flowers that grow there. I know that even if I'm not there to see them they are going to come up out of the ground in the spring. They are going to grow and they will be beautiful. If I'm there to see them it will be a gift, a joy, and I'm looking forward to it. But even if I'm not there they will be. Others will enjoy them. I helped to put them there, and that gives me a special feeling. I can't quite put it into words — a different kind of hoping?"

17
I Was a Stranger

The stranger who shows kindness in another's trouble
gives courage that comes flowing out of tears of joy.

WHEN ONE is very sick one is often surprised by the kindness and generosity of people in all walks of life. Family and friends who love and care sustain and support one in inestimable ways. There is another kindness, however, that one experiences on quite a different level. It comes at the most unexpected times and from the most unexpected people: usually complete strangers, sometimes slight acquaintances. This kindness is often the most moving and touching of all the experiences connected with dying.

One of my earliest experiences came about soon after surgery, when I was spending a great deal of time in bed trying to cope with the effects of chemotherapy.

The telephone rang and I was told that a man whom I had never met had heard about my illness through his wife and wanted to do something for me. He had been told of my love of music, and he proposed to set up a complete sound system in my bedroom. And that is what he did. It was more than three years ago now and the system is playing as I write. I don't think that man will ever really understand what he did that day. He installed costly equipment that I could never have purchased, giving me hours and hours of listening joy that overcame many times of weakness and pain. But the most precious gift was and still is the underlying, totally unexpected, basic human kindness and generosity: I was a stranger.

There was a lady in the hospital unit who, unable to speak or move, could still indicate with her eyes when a favourite piece of music was played on her bedside radio. I often think of her.

Other events crowd into my mind, each one uniquely moving, some to laughter, some to tears. All are the precious gifts of caring strangers.

Late one night the doorbell rang. There on the doorstep, white-faced, strained (fortified by quite a number of stiff drinks), obviously petrified but equally determined, stood a local shopkeeper with whom I had dealt for some years. He came in awkwardly and thrust a folder into my hands. It contained the names of some faith healers whose lectures he had attended. He blurted out, "It was hard to come. My wife thinks I'm crazy; she doesn't even know I'm here. She thinks I'm still working. I nearly didn't make it — walked all the way up the hill. But I couldn't live with myself if I didn't at least try to find some help for you. That's why I've come. I can't just stand by and watch you die without trying to help."

Christmas came, and friends visited with gifts, and some who were afraid stayed away. A young woman I knew telephoned to say that she had cooked something for me and could she "bring it 'round." She arrived wearing the attire of the Yoga Institute where she lived and worked, a white robe with a saffron scarf at her neck. She was weighed down by shopping bags and bundles. "Everyone decided that they would like to do something for you this Christmas," she told me, "so we 'gave you Sunday.' We all worked all day, cooking and baking, even the children."

Her shopping bags seemed bottomless. "This is a fruit cake and here are eight more just like it. This is a banana loaf; there are six of them in this bag. These are the cookies [various varieties neatly packed in several boxes]. Here are the candies and the little gingerbread men. The children made those; see how they inserted the raisins for eyes, noses, and mouths, and the buttons down the front. They were so busy and so happy doing it for you." On and on it went. The table groaned under the burden. I pictured all those people working away, anticipating the pleasure they would give to a person they would never see. Her voice went on, "Of course, you may want to use some of them as presents, but you will have enough to serve guests and people who call to see you during the holidays as well." They had given me selfless, generous gifts of time, energy, and precious resources that would enable me in turn to have the pleasure of giving, something which that year had seemed impossible and which they, the strangers, had thought about.

Looking back over these four years, I could write of many incidents. With cheery smiles and encouraging banter, those oft-berated taxi drivers go out of their way to help me in and out in all kinds of weather. When I shopped at the local supermarket, frail little old ladies in the check-out line insisted on unloading my cart at the wicket, all the time chatting friendly, motherly words of kindness. A young girl, totally unknown, stopped me on the street and asked if I had far to go because it would be no trouble for her to drive me in her car.

The last incident occurred only a few days ago. I was coming home from the hospital, climbing awkwardly out of the taxi at the door, collar and bandages as usual supporting fragile cancerous bones. Suddenly beside me there stood a little man, a passerby. I used to see him when I walked our little dog. He lives somewhere in a nearby apartment block. We had smiled and nodded, never more. This day he came over to me and said, "I've watched you for a long time wearing that thing. You aren't getting any better, are you? Do you mind if I ask what's wrong?" I smiled to try and reassure him, replying, "No, I am not getting better. It is cancer." There was a silence. I saw his eyes cloud. He muttered awkwardly and haltingly, "Listen, you've probably got all kinds of people helping you, I know. But if you ever need anything, anything at all, I want you to know it's alright to ask — I mean I'd really be glad." With that he stumbled away.

I made my way into the elevator. Tears filled my eyes. I could not see. Those tears were tears of joy, the gift of yet another stranger. And then through the tears I smiled. That kind-hearted little man — I didn't even know his name.

123

18
Joy

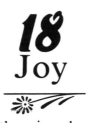

And where there is sadness — joy![13]

DYING OF cancer does not always mean times of sadness and gloom. Sometimes laughter and fun come to relieve even the worst moments. I witnessed this many times in the hospital ward and I know it in my own life now.

There is also the wonderful paradox of joy in the pain. C.S. Lewis described it when he wrote of his wife's time of dying. He said, "It is incredible how much happiness, how much gaiety we sometimes had together even after all hope had gone."[24]

The English lady who kept the diary of her illness and dying and who described her excruciating pain so vividly was still able to write during the last summer of her life, "I feel suffused by love, bubbling and running over with it, until it runs out of my ears. I can only think of this as one of the happiest summers in memory yet now I can't swim, walking grows increasingly difficult, my stomach grows, and none of my clothes will fit."[25]

I understand what she was feeling. There is overwhelming appreciation and gratitude for the ones who really love and care, the ones who have stayed the course and who are always present when you need them. When a person looks at you and loves, you are no longer ugly and unclean with disease, and each day seems a precious gift to be cherished and savoured to the full.

Seated in the chair, the corners of your lips
drawn tight, plumb my eyes like a well,

127

Is it politeness, is it duty, or
Unfailing love that . . . binds me to you still?

Each morning you are more sallow, more tired.
As I comb out your hair I find it breaks off.
Your arm has dried up like a vine. On your neck
lumps of cancer are swelling. Through the window
the sky is blue, the mountain slopes indifferent.

Today you feel no pain. I sit beside you
on the bed and hold your coffee cup. In place
of little breasts are purplish pustules.
I have this dream that you will not go away,
that we will remain together one decade more.

My love, my sceptre, who weighs eighty pounds!
What is there to say?   Blessed be this day,
for the spirit still flickers in your ravaged body,
for your eyes, pastel-grey, are still beautiful,
and even like this life is marvellous, never better.[26]

Afterword

AT THE time that I finished writing this little book it seemed unlikely that I would be alive to see its publication.

But now several years have passed and I am still here. The cancer remains. But the symptoms are controlled and I am able to function in a limited way. Life is still good and precious and I like to think that my continuing survival, against all the odds, may bring some hope to others in similar circumstances.

I am in the country for much of the time but continue to work among the dying patients and their families by means of the telephone.

My life is constantly enriched by the close contact with so many people who are facing the challenges of their illness with great courage, faith and hope. They, and those who love and support them, bear witness to the fact that, despite the inevitable pain and suffering, grave illness *can* bring special gifts and opportunities that enable us to find deeper meaning in our lives, and lead to that final sense of peace and acceptance.

For me the journey continues. No one can predict for how long. Life has to be lived one day at a time. But I am grateful for the joy, the hopes and the challenges that each new day brings. Once more I can truly say

> For all that has been — Thanks!
> To all that shall be — Yes!

Sources of Quotations

p. vii Dag Hammarskjöld, *Markings* (London: Faber & Faber, 1964), p. 87.

1. Rabindranath Ragore, *Stray Birds*. (CCXCIII). Copyright © 1916, The Macmillan Co., renewed 1944, Tagore Rabindranath.
2. Viktor Frankl, *Man's Search for Meaning* (Boston: Beacon Press, 1963).
3. Rabindranath Tagore, *A Tagore Reader: Poems Old and New* (New York: the Macmillan Co, 1961), p. 352.
4. Suzanne D. Field, "A Message," unpublished poem.
5. Rabindranath Tagore, *Fireflies* (New York: Macmillan Publishing Co., Inc., 1976), p. 268.
6. T.S. Eliot, *Collected Poems, 1909-1935* (New York: Harcourt, Brace & World, Inc., 1934). Copyright © 1930, 1958 by T.S. Eliot; copyright 1934, 1936 by Harcourt, Brace & World, Inc.
7. C.S. Lewis, *A Grief Observed* (New York: Seabury Press, 1963).
8. Diana Gault, *A Journey* (London: Chatto and Windus, 1968).
9. Tagore, *Fireflies*, p. 69.
10. Edward Fitzgerald, The Rubáiyát of Omar Khayyam (New York: Avon books, 1968).
11. Hammarskjöld, *Markings*, p. 175.
12. Tagore, *Fireflies*, p. 139.
13. *Ibid.*, p. 243.
14. Claudia Behrendt, extract from a diary, unpublished.
15. Anonymous, "Death in the First Person," *American Journal of Nursing* (Feb. 1970).
16. André Gide, *Springs of Hope*, edited by E. Hettinger, translated by Peter M. Daly (New York: Herder and Herder, 1971).
17. I Cor. 13:12.
18. Tagore, *Fireflies*, p. 231.
19. Vittorio Alfieri.
20. *Macbeth*, act IV, sc. 3, lines 210-211.
21. Colin Murray Parkes, *Bereavement: Studies of Grief in Adult Life* (New York: International Universities Press, 1973).
22. Emily Dickinson, "Hope Is the Thing with Feathers," in *Selected Poems and Letters* (Garden City, NY: Doubleday, 1959), p. 79.
23. St. Francis of Assisi, Prayer.
24. Lewis, *Grief Observed*.
25. Gault, *Journey*.
26. George Faludy, "Love Poems to Her Dying," in *East and West*, translated by Andrew Faludy (Toronto: Hounslow Press, 1963).